A Little Bit of Something Beats a Whole Lot of Nothing

A 30 Day Guide to Your New Healthy Habits

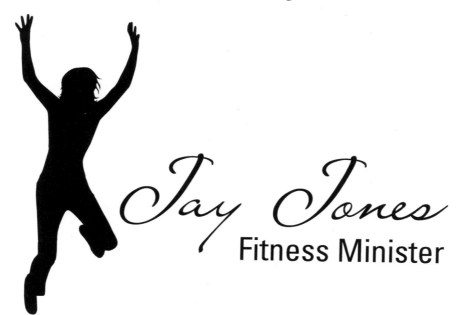

Jay Jones
Fitness Minister

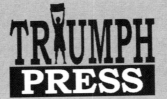

Triumph Press is a resource for those who have the passion to tell their life-stories and change the world. If you have a true and inspiring story to share, visit *www.TriumphPress.com* to learn how we can help you publish and join our library of inspirational books.

Dedication

I would like to thank God for the grace, divine influence and supernatural blessings to allow me to complete this "Little bit of something" to be of service to you.

I dedicate this, my first book, to my very best friend, number one cheerleader, and my partner for life, my wife April Jones. Without your continued encouragement, motivation, and sometimes aggervation (to keep me on task) this book would have remained another "good idea" that didn't see the light of day! Thanks for the one LIFE stand baby!

I would also like to dedicate this book to YOU! I know your trying to do the very best you can with the resources, time, and talents you have but things don't to seem to be turning out the way you would like. Well this book was designed to help you cut through the clutter and reclaim your freedom, fitness and future by simply doing a little bit of something as opposed to a whole lot of nothing regarding your earthly temple! I pray that you allow these words to fall upon fertile soil so they can bud, blossom, and bear the fruit of a new healthy habit into your life!

Table of Contents

"Nothing is as hard as it looks; everything is more rewarding than you expect; and if anything can go right it will and at the best possible moment."

~ John C Maxwell

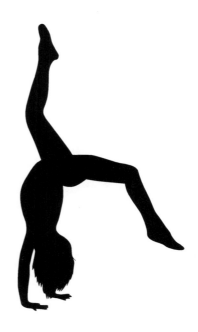

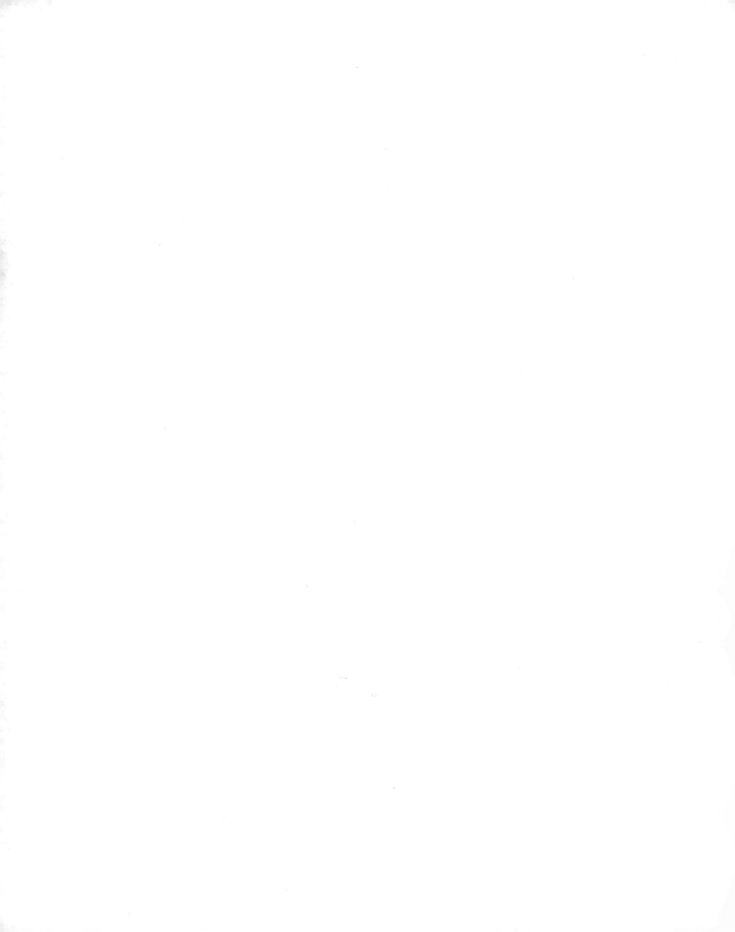

ON YOUR MARK, GET SET

"We are what we repeatedly do.
Excellence then, is not an act, but a habit."
~ Aristotle.

How many times have you tried to start a new healthy habit and failed? Have you become frustrated and irritated with your own lack of discipline and inability to change? If you are truly ready to create a new healthy habit and gain greater mental clarity in just 30 days, I highly suggest you continue reading.

The whole point of changing your habits is to change your lifestyle, which will ultimately change your life. That's exactly what this book is intended to accomplish… change your life! You'll learn how to create small victories everyday by accomplishing very doable physical feats and nutritional milestones, such as touching your toes, taking a five minute walk and eating incrementally larger portions of fruits and vegetables while slowly removing processed food from the bulk of your fuel source. The idea is to master something small and build on each success until you make the rest of your life the best of your life… one new healthy habit at a time!

I wrote this book because I wanted to share more than a decade of hands on experience I have training, teaching, and inspiring people to change their life through the power of doing just a little bit of something everyday toward building the body, business, or best life they desire and deserve. I know firsthand how "life" can happen to our very best intentions. I was a promising football player but my dreams of becoming a professional were derailed by a career ending broken neck. I not only needed to rehabilitate my body, but my entire value system had to be rebuilt. That took patience, perseverance and definitely the cultivation of healthy new habits! I used the exact same techniques and strategies that you will learn in this book to change my life and then the lives of my clients. I hope you will allow them to change your life as well!

I wanted to write and design the most valuable book possible, so my publisher and I created a workbook to give you the greatest transformational experience, as opposed to simply being educated. The workbook is written with a powerful quote to introduce you to your exercise (or movement) each day, for the next 30 days. You will also have an opportunity to Journal the Journey to help you internalize the lessons you will learn and galvanize your new healthy habits.

I pray this book penetrates the most persistent doubt and excuses you have used to prevent you from achieving what you really want for yourself and your loved ones. We can never solve a problem with the same information used to create the problem; we must heighten our awareness and learn new strategies in order to evolve. A Little Bit of Something Beats a whole lot of Nothing gives you the opportunity to incrementally build your body and brain so you can create solutions through evolution! Are you ready to grow... then let's GO!

A Little Bit of Something...

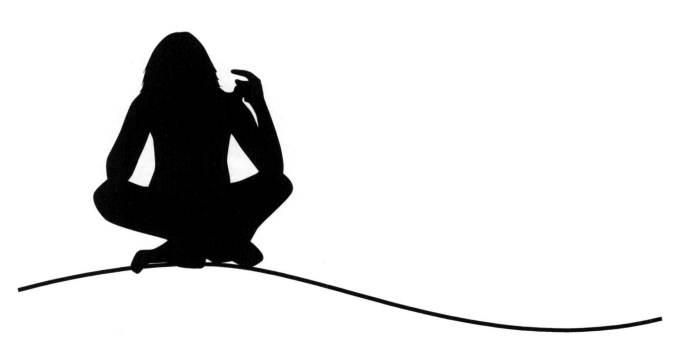

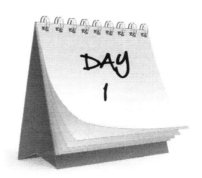

"Bravery is not a quality of the body.
It is of the soul."
~ Mahatma Gandhi

Today's little bit of something is a 10 minute walk in your neighborhood, office complex, favorite park or anywhere you can walk 5 minutes out and 5 minutes back. You are encouraged to do more if possible but not required.

Your Fitness Footnote for today is to be BRAVE!

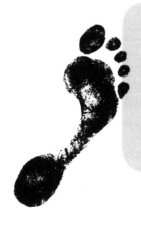

Change takes courage. It requires that you be disciplined and determined not to sacrifice what you want most for what you want now. Change requires patience, perseverance and pitbull-like persistence. But most of all, it requires you to be BRAVE- to do what needs to be done in spite of the fear, discomfort or time commitment. You must be Brave to carve out a new healthy habit in the next 30 days!

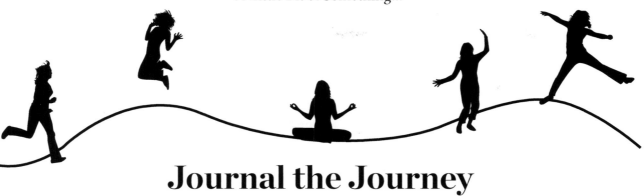

Journal the Journey

Recall and write down the last time you had to be BRAVE! Struggle creates amnesia... it makes us forget that we have already overcome greater adversity than doing a little bit of something every day to build your brain and body!

11

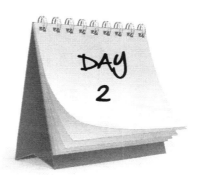

"And let us not be weary in well doing:
for in due season we shall reap, if we faint not."
~ Galatians 6:9

Today's little bit of something is simply touching your toes, or as close as you can get to them, 5 times from a standing position. Start by standing tall and then bend at the waist making sure to keep your legs straight and then touch your toes. Hold the bottom position for 2 seconds. Do not bounce. Now return to your starting position. Repeat 4 more times. You are encouraged but not required to take another 10 minute walk after you stretch.

Your fitness footnote for today is to FOCUS ON THE FUNDAMENTALS!

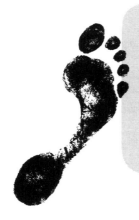

We live in a very high tech but low touch society, so we must focus on the fundamentals in order to reap the benefits of a strong, healthy mind and body. Drink lots of water, eat fresh organic (homegrown is always best) fruits and veggies, move responsibly (exercise), and most importantly, control and minimize the deadly disease maker, stress! Focusing on the fundamentals is key to developing your new healthy habit.

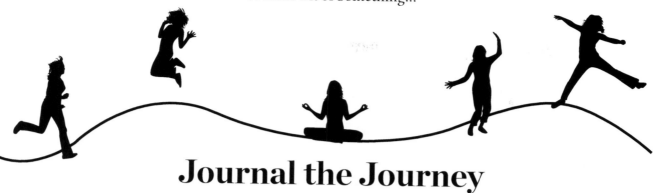

Journal the Journey

Write down three basic things you promise to do TODAY for yourself! You can take the stairs instead of the elevator/escalator, a cat-nap to help rejuvenate yourself, park further from the front door wherever you go, sit still outside for five minutes and mediate. WHATEVER you decide to do to get back to the fundamentals, write it down to make it real!

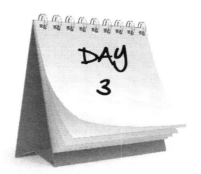

"Never let your head hang down. Never give up and sit down and grieve. Find another way. And don't pray when it rains if you don't pray when the sun shines."
~ Leroy Satchel Paige

Today's little bit of something is doing 5 floor push-ups. You remember the good ole push-up, don't you? Just lay down on your stomach, place your palms flat on the ground right next to your chest and tighten your core as you exhale and push yourself off the floor...keeping your body rigid and at a perfect angle (no drooping in the middle). Go back down... all the way to the floor... rest for 3 seconds and repeat 4 more times. Remember to keep your core tight, inhale as you go down and exhale as you push yourself up forcefully. You are encouraged, as always, to do more if you can. Continue to walk and touch those toes as well.

Your fitness footnote for today is all about FORGIVENESS!

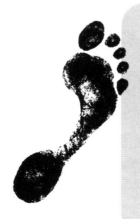

I'm not just talking about the traditional idea of you forgiving someone else, but I'm referring specifically to forgiving yourself! In the past, you may not have made the best decisions when it came to your nutrition or exercise... forgive yourself. You may not be proud of where you are right now physically... forgive yourself. You may struggle with the discipline it takes to do even a little bit of something.... forgive yourself. Do not beat yourself up, be ashamed, or quit! Acknowledge your mistakes, forgive yourself and move on with a renewed faith and fearlessness toward your goal. Forgiveness is essential to developing your new healthy habit!

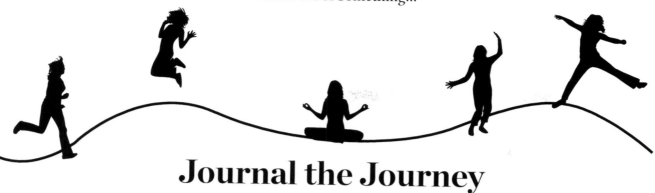

Journal the Journey

Grab a piece of paper and write down three things you need to forgive yourself for; then forgive yourself and (safely) burn the paper you wrote on! The process of physically burning the burdens will immediately lighten your load and intensify the feeling of forgiveness. Be honest, as always, when writing what you want to forgive yourself about... the more sincere the forgiveness the greater the feeling of relief and rejuvenation! Then write on this Journal the Journey page how it feels to be forgiven.

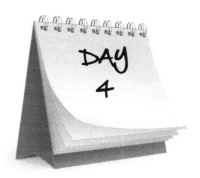

"Don't say you don't have enough time. You have exactly the same number of hours per day that were given to Martin Luther King, Jesus, Harriet Tubman, Mother Teresa, Leonardo da Vinci, Malcolm X, and Albert Einstein."

~ *Jay Jones, Fitness Minister*

Today's little bit of something is doing 10 old fashion squats! We all know what a squat is, but many of us aren't sure how to do it properly. Although squats are amazing for building strong, toned legs and butts, if done wrong they can possibly injure your knees. So let's go over the squat… I want you to imagine standing with your back against a glass wall. Now imagine sliding down that wall and as your knees bend, push your hips back (imagine breaking the glass with your butt) as you keep your back straight and chest up. Inhale as you go down and exhale as you push back up to the starting position. Be sure that your knees don't jut out over your toes, but keep them in line with your ankles. This is the mistake which causes the most injuries in the squat exercise. Now repeat 9 more times. You are encouraged to do more, as always.

Your fitness footnote for today focuses on TIME!

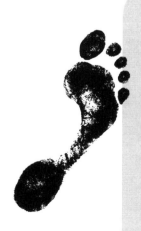

If good health is our greatest asset, then time is the most precious commodity we own. We can spend time, but we cannot buy any more of it. We are all allotted the same amount of hours every day as the richest or the poorest person on the planet. What are you doing with your precious time? Are you building or destroying the life you want to truly live? Are you feeding or fighting stress and disease? Are you choosing life or death with the way you spend your time? Time is much too valuable to waste or throw away so make sure you are building the body and the life you deserve by investing your time in activities that will yield a positive return. Good time management will be essential in developing your new healthy habit in 30 days.

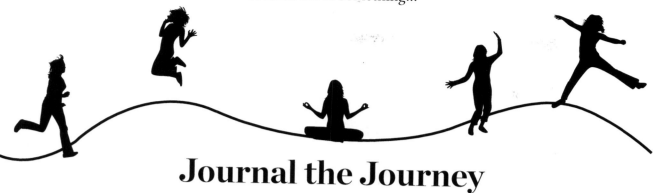

Journal the Journey

Recall and write down three areas or activities where you invest most of your time (outside of work). Now honestly ask yourself, is this time investment building the body, business, or the very best life you deserves? If the answer is anything other than "yes," then decide to re-invest your time into things that edify your physical, financial and mental well being TODAY.

"When things are bad, we take comfort in the thought that they could always get worse. And when they are, we find hope in the thought that things are so bad they have to get better."
~ *Malcolm S Forbes*

Today's little bit of something is simply to drink 8 glasses of water. We are comprised of 50% to 60% water so it makes sense that we need water not only to survive, but to thrive and live fully. Without proper hydration, our digestion, energy, mental faculties and overall health is compromised. We tend to eat more, age faster and encounter more inflammation when we are dehydrated. It is recommended that we drink 8 glasses of water a day to maintain healthy hydration, so down a little bit of something by drinking that many glasses today.

Your fitness footnote for today is to have HOPE.

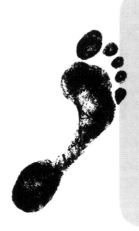

Change is challenging! It will test you physically, mentally and spiritually. But in the face of all the challenges that change provides, there is a powerful force that will always work in your favor... HOPE. You must always remain hopeful in the face of any adversity. You must always have the audacity to believe you can conquer any obstacles, physical or mental, that threaten to prevent you from achieving your objective. It is hope that will keep you afloat when your will begins to waver and sink. Stay hopeful through the challenges and watch your new healthy habit become a reality.

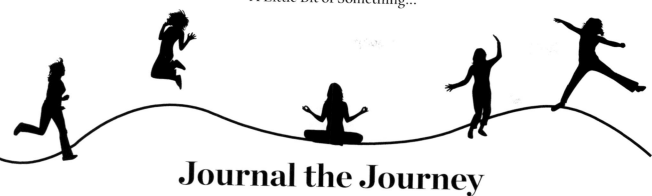

Journal the Journey

Recall and write down a situation you believed was hopeless. Now look at what you wrote and re-imagine that same situation infused with hope and a great expectation of success. Hope is a state of mind, as opposed to a tangible, touchable thing, so you can harness the power of hope by simply changing your perspective of the problem... give it a try right now!

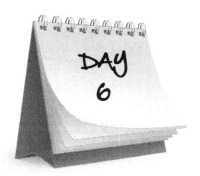

"If you are too busy to laugh, you are too busy."
~ Proverb

Today's little bit of something is simply getting down on the ground, flat on your belly, then getting back up into a complete standing position. Now do 7 more... for a total of 8. It may seem simple, but this little move engages every major muscle group in your body. You are encouraged to do as many as you can, if 8 is not enough. A little extra something is always recommended but not necessary.

Your fitness footnote for today is to LAUGH IT UP!

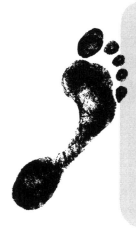

Laughter is amazing medicine. It is an unbridled expression of joy and contentment; if only for a fleeting moment. We laugh when we feel good and we feel good when we laugh. Laughter reduces anxiety which causes us to minimize the disease producing problem we all have called stress! When we smile and laugh through a great workout, it actually helps our physical performance as well as our recovery time and mental state of mind. Watch a funny movie, visit a comedy club, download a joke of the day podcast or simply hang out with a funny friend. Laughter will be an intricate part of developing your new healthy habit.

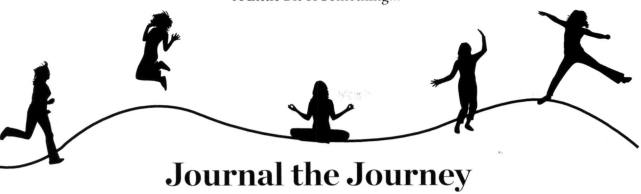

Journal the Journey

Laughing is medication! Seriously! When was the last time you laughed so hard you cried? Recall and write down three of the funniest moments you've had in the past few months. It could have been a show, a comedian or just something in your daily life that made you laugh out loud. Relax, re-live and re-laugh at the moment all over again as you write it down.

"I am sorry for the inconvenience, but this is a revolution."
~ Malcolm X

Your little bit of something for today is to hold a 30 second plank. A plank is exactly what it sounds like. Your body is going to mimic a hard wooden board. You need to get down on your hands and knees. Now I want you to brace your upper body on your forearms and elbows while you extend your legs out as if you were about to do a push-up. The only point of contact on the floor should be your forearm, elbows and toes. Your back should be nice and flat; no peaks or valleys. Breathe normally as you hold this position for 30 seconds without falling to the floor. The plank is a tremendously efficient core strengthener and mental exercise. You are encouraged to do 2 rounds of 30 second planks but only one is REQUIRED.

Your Fitness Footnote for today is to be REVOLUTIONARY!

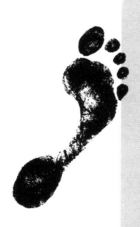

Being healthy in a sick society is a revolutionary act! The huge pharmaceutical "cartels," global fast food peddlers, and greedy healthcare and insurance corporations all want to keep us addicted to their pills, potions, powders and promises in order to fatten their pockets! The current American "Death Style" has the U.S. ranked as the second (closely behind Mexico) most obese nation in the world! Our current obesity epidemic affects every area of our lives - including the way we socialize, exercise and prioritize our health and wellness. In order to reclaim your fitness and freedom, you must be revolutionary in your thinking and actions. Be revolutionary by being committed to educating yourself and the ones you love about being fit. Be revolutionary by eating fresh, locally grown (whenever possible) organic fruits and vegetables. Keep your body and brain strong through responsible movement. Revolutionary action is essential to creating your new healthy habit.

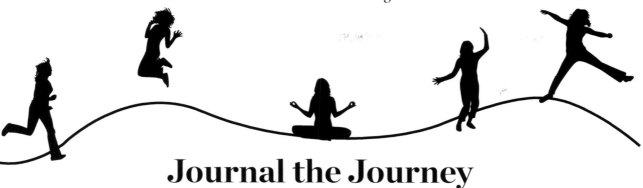

Journal the Journey

What revolutionary person motivates you? Who in history or in your life inspires you to be David to the Goliath in you may be facing? Whose story of action in the face of adversity gives you the courage and resilience to be revolutionary in your daily thoughts and actions? Recall and write down the person or people you are fighting for by reading this book ... and be revolutionary in your commitment to complete a little bit of something every day!

23

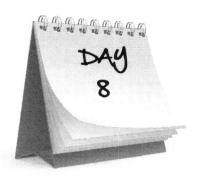

> ## *"When you visualize, then you materialize. If you've been there in the mind you'll go there in the body."*
> ## *~ Denis Waitley*

Your little bit of something for today is to eat 2 servings of fresh vegetables. 80% of your fitness goals are a direct result of your diet and nutrition so it is extremely important that you feed your body what it needs to succeed. Empty calories are available everywhere we go and if we are not careful, we will fill up on foods that only serve to make us sick and dependent on "drugs" to make us feel better. When we eat foods designed specifically for human consumption (food that appears in nature), we grow stronger, smarter and enjoy a healthier, happier, longer life. As always, you are encouraged to eat more than the 2 servings, but not required.

Your Fitness Footnote for today is to VISUALIZE THE POSSIBILITIES!

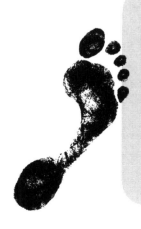

In life, we must have a vision in order to achieve anything of significance. A vision of your ideal body, ideal health and ideal reality will help you remain disciplined and encouraged. Visualize how a new level of fitness, energy and intellect will improve your relationships and overall quality of life! The possibilities are endless on how much value your new healthy habit will provide for you if you can visualize it! See what you want to be... and then become it! Visualize completing this 30 day Healthy Habit program and watch your new healthy habits change your life.

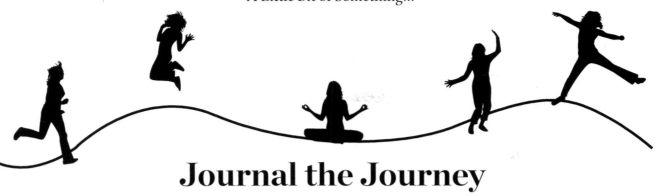

Journal the Journey

Visualization is key to manifestation! Say it out loud... visualization is key to manifestation! Say it one more time, visualization is key to manifestation! The only place you can ever perform perfectly is in your thoughts. When you visualize whatever you're about to engage in, your brain literally goes through the same motions as if you were actually engaging in the activity for real. Your breathing and heart rate also respond to the visualization as if you were actually experiencing the event. This "pre-experience" or "perfect practice" of the situation allows you to visualize the outcome you desire and expect it to turn out exactly as you have already experienced it. Try it right now! Take five minutes to recall and write down an upcoming challenge in your life (job interview, big meeting, presentation, workout session, etc.) and then take five more minutes to actually visualize yourself doing it perfectly and getting the exact results you want. The more detailed and specific you are with the visualization, the more powerful the positive programming. Practice this powerful technique at least once a day for the next 22 days!

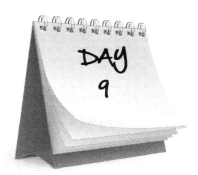

DAY 9

*"The ultimate measure of a man is not where he stands
in moments of comfort and convenience, but where he stands
at times of challenge and controversy."*
~ *Martin Luther King*

Your little bit of something for today is to do an Air-bike for 30 seconds. The Air-bike is one of the most effective CORE (not just ab) exercises you can do anytime and anywhere. Start by lying flat on your back. Put your hands behind your head and imagine there is a tennis ball between your chin and chest. Take your outstretched legs and drive your right knee into your chest while extending your left leg straight out, six inches off the ground then alternate "peddling" by extending and retracting your legs in and out - six inches off the ground for 30 seconds. As always, you are encouraged to do more if you are able but it is not required.

Your Fitness Footnote for today is to CHALLENGE YOURSELF!

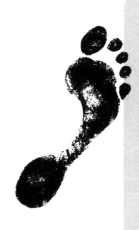

Without challenge, there is no change in life... period! Many of us would be extremely excited if we could have the money we need, the health and fitness we desire and the lifestyle we dream about without having to get uncomfortable to acquire it. We may be able to endure adversities for a short time, but as life begins to happen to us, our ability to endure the challenge of maintaining our commitment begins to run out and we resort back to our old, comfortable way of doing things. When that happens, we sacrifice what we want MOST for what we want NOW. In other words, our desire to avoid challenge and remain comfortable overrides our desire to face the challenge in order to benefit from the changes. As a result, we remain unhealthy, under-paid, and generally unsatisfied with our situation. I want you to decide today that you are up for the CHALLENGE of changing your life! You CAN and WILL do this by simply doing a little bit of something toward to your health and wellness every day to insure you develop your new healthy habit in 30 days!

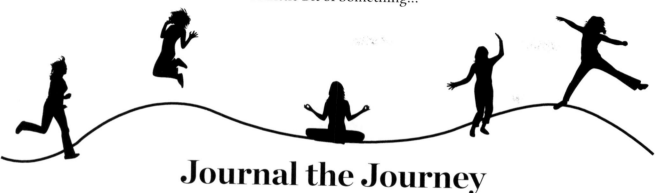

Journal the Journey

Challenge requires you to get uncomfortable in order to change. You cannot solve a problem with the exact same knowledge used to create the problem! Something has to change; your intellect, environment, or others involvement has to change in order to evolve. What challenge can you conquer to push yourself into the life you desire and deserve today? Recall and write down something RIGHT NOW that you've put off, pushed off, and neglected to do because you don't FEEL like it. Once it's written, if it's doable right now... do it right now! Make the call, order the course, take that jog, schedule that doctor appointment, eat those delicious vegetables or WHATEVER you need to do to challenge yourself enough to achieve the life you desire and deserve! Do it now.... I'll wait!

27

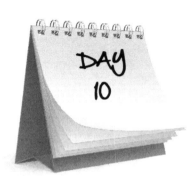

DAY 10

" I am the GREATEST,' I said that even before I knew I was!"
~ Muhammed Ali

Your little bit of something for today is to do Jumping Jacks for 30 seconds. If your joints will not allow you to jump, you can modify by stepping from side to side as you arch your arms above your head and return to a normal standing position when your arms are at your side. You are encouraged to do as much as your body and mind will allow if 30 seconds is not enough. Try doing 2 rounds of 30 seconds if you can.

Your Fitness Footnote for today is DON'T BE GOOD, BE GREAT!

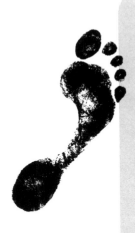

Each and every one of us has some form of greatness within. It may be locked under layers of doubt, fear, excuses and neglect, but it is still there, waiting for the moment in your life when something external or internal awakens it! But the enemy of great is and has always been... good. Most of us will go through life and good will be "good enough." We will settle on good because you don't have to work as hard to be good. You don't have to get as uncomfortable to be good. You don't have to be as patient to be good. So we forgo our greatness. We allow the greatness in us to be bought by a few dollars, forgotten for a few moments of pleasure or stolen by a slick talker who wants to misuse and abuse our greatness. We allow our greatness to get old, fat and uninspired because good was good enough. Don't allow that to happen to you! I want you to employ the Ali Strategy and tell yourself "I am the greatest!" Don't just say it, but believe it and expect it. When asked, don't say, "I'm having a good day," say "I'm having a GREAT day!" "I'm not feeling good, I'm feeling GREAT!" "My business is not just doing good, it's doing GREAT!" Greatness is your natural state, so never settle for good when you were born to be GREAT! Your internal greatness will certainly help you develop your new healthy habit in 30 days.

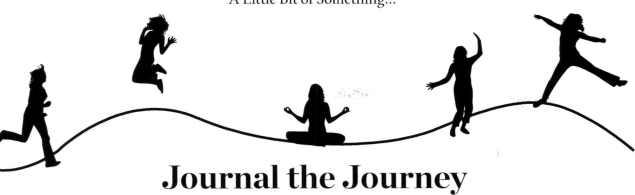

Journal the Journey

What does good mean to you? What does great mean to you? Write down these two questions and honestly answer them. Remember, there is no wrong answer only an authentic one. When you define something in your own words, you demonstrate your understanding of it. Now recall and write down two instances or situations where you know you settled for being "good" as opposed to "great," and then write what you would do differently today. The good only becomes great when you realize what needs to be done!

29

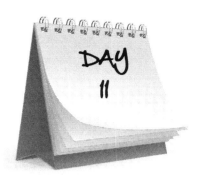

"Teamwork makes the dream work!"
~ Jay Jones, Fitness Minister

Your little bit of something for today is to spend 20 minutes outdoors doing something physical. You can walk, play basketball, cut your grass, detail your car or simply stretch in the sun. Being outside can help improve your mood, mentality and muscles. Going to the gym has become one of America's favorite pastimes. We spend so much time in these "artificial environments" that we forget that they are just that... artificial environments. Fluorescent lights, stale and recycled air, germ filled machines and crowded locker rooms pale in comparison to sunshine, fresh flowing air and abundant space to explore. You are encouraged to spend more time communing in nature, but 20 minutes is sufficient today.

Your Fitness Footnote today is BUILD YOUR TEAM!

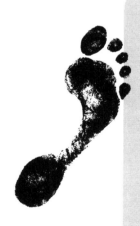

No man (or woman) is an island! This old adage simply means we need another individual, group, community or team in order to manifest our dream! There is indeed power in numbers. Hollywood celebrities depend on a team of people from agents to managers to publicist and coaches, to make them successful. Corporate tycoons depend on a team of advisors and strategists to make them millions and even world class athletes have a personal team of trainers, nutritionists and a sport psychologist to keep them performing at their peak. Who comprises your team? Is your team helping or hurting your chances to be successful? Your team should help you stay focused, inspired, educated, motivated and accountable in order for you to maximize the benefits of your new healthy habit and lifestyle. People with training partners are more successful when it comes to maintaining their new healthy habits compared with those who don't.

Remove or minimize any negative elements from your team and constantly evaluate if you and your teammates are all working toward the same goals and objectives. Knowing that teamwork makes the dream work will be important for you to create your new healthy habit in 30 days.

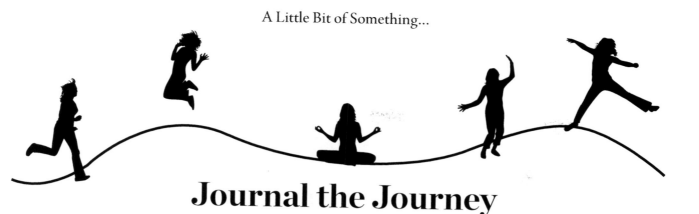

Journal the Journey

Pretend you are the coach of a world champion basketball team and need to assemble your starting five players. Each player will have to possess a certain skill set unique to his/her position on the team. Your life mirrors the imaginary basketball team. You also need to recruit and build a lineup of people that can bring unique gifts and talents together for the sake of creating a winning team! Recall and write down the name of the person you would consider the MVP (Most Valuable Person) of your team and why. Next, recall and write down two things that make you a good team member.

DAY
12

"The world belongs to the self-confident risk taker,
who is bright enough to believe he can accomplish anything,
and tough enough to persist until he proves it."
~ *Steve Siebol*

Your little bit of something for today is doing mountain climbers for 20 seconds. You may not know what this exercise is, but I am certain you have seen it done before. To start, get down on your hands and knees and then move into a push-up position. Instead of doing a push-up, you are going to alternate "climbing" by driving one knee at a time into your chest (keep your foot off the ground when you bring it into your chest) while planting your back foot into the ground. Keep your back flat and breathe in through your nose and out through your mouth. You are always encouraged to do more than 20 seconds if you are able.

Your fitness footnote for today is to be TOUGH!

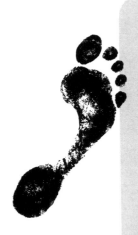

We are truly living in the best of times and possibly the worst of times. Our technology revolution has put the entire catalog of human knowledge at our fingertips; providing us with the answer to any question we can possibly ask in mere seconds... that's pretty good. But that same technology offers so many choices and so much information that many of us simply get "overloaded" and do nothing... that's not so good! We lose our drive, creativity and, perhaps most importantly, we start to lose our toughness! Toughness is defined by our ability to endure periods of hardship and difficulties both physically and mentally in order to overcome or achieve something. In past years people have had to endure tremendous physical and mental hardships in order to create our current way of life. The level of toughness they displayed on a daily basis kept them strong, creative and resilient. Are you tough enough to endure the challenges of your new healthy change? Can you summon the mental and physical toughness necessary to reap the rewards of your new healthy habit? Yes you are; and yes you can! Tough times don't last but tough people do! You must tap into your internal toughness tank in order to maximize your new healthy habit in 30 days.

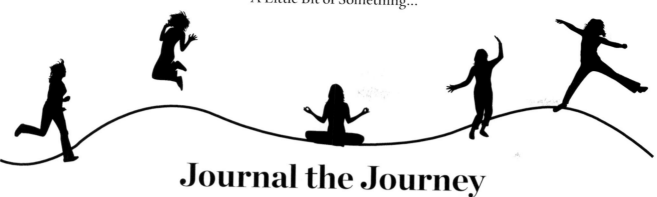

Journal the Journey

Toughness is defined as being strong and durable... not easily broken. Can you recall times in your life when you demonstrated your toughness? Write down three moments (a workout, a tough assignment, a competitive contest, a traumatic event, etc.) where you felt strong and durable... not easily broken. Review the list and apply the same level of toughness you have already displayed to whatever obstacles that are on your current path to your new healthy habit!

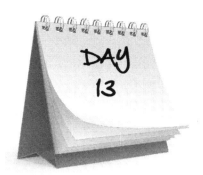

*"Now faith is the assurance of things hoped for,
the conviction of things not seen."*
~ Hebrews 11:1

Your little bit of something for today is to dance to two of your favorite up-tempo songs back to back. Believe it or not, dancing is one of the best cardio exercises you can do. Don't believe me? Turn up your favorite dance tunes and "bust a move" for the entire two songs! You will get your blood flowing, heart going and endurance growing! When you dance, you burn calories, increase oxygen in your body and reduce stress. So put on your dancing shoes and "shake a tail feather." You are encouraged to dance as much as you can but two of your favorite songs back to back will be enough today.

Your Fitness Footnote for today is to have a little FAITH!

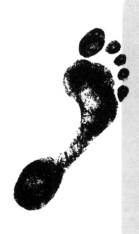

Billions of people across the globe have a belief in something greater than themselves. They believe that there is a force, energy, presence or spirit that has a supernatural influence on our daily affairs that cannot be explained. This phenomenon is what some may call faith. Faith is a powerful motivator that can help people achieve extraordinary things. Mountains can move, giants can fall and lives can be changed if we truly believe and have a little faith that it is possible! When we attach our faith to our fitness, we can experience the same supernatural power to overcome obstacles, remain disciplined and reap the rewards of staying committed to change. When the pressure of life begins to weigh heavy on us and we lose focus on our fitness, we can employ our faith to give us the courage and conviction to live the life we were created achieve. Faith has played and continues to play a vital role in the lives of billions of people worldwide. Allow your faith to fortify your new healthy habit in 30 days.

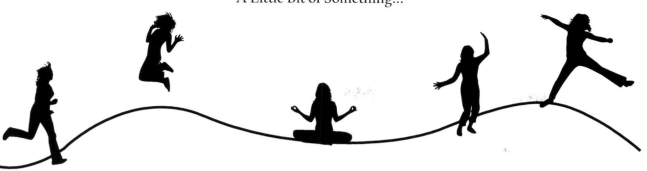

Journal the Journey

Our mind can be our greatest ally or our supreme adversary. Our perspective and values influence our thoughts and behavior so it is important to manage and balance the external pressures of life with an internal value system based on something more substantial. Recall and write down three moments when you relied on your faith to help motivate, activate and generate the courage and conviction you needed to achieve something important. Just thinking about these powerful demonstrations of faith in action from your past should inspire more courage and conviction in your daily struggles.

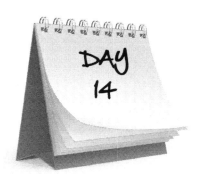

DAY 14

"Breathe. Let go. And remind yourself that this very moment is the only one you know you have for sure."
~ *Oprah Winfrey*

Your little bit of something for today will focus on your posture and balance. We age from the ground up, meaning our lower body strength, speed and flexibility erodes before our upper body. As a result, we run a greater risk of injury through slips, falls or a combination of the two. We must build and maintain our temples from the ground up. I want you to try an exercise called a knee hug. If your balance is compromised in any way, please stand by a wall or something you can grab and regain your balance if necessary. To do this exercise stand nice and tall, with your chest out and shoulders pressed down and back (shoulder blades relaxed). Next, balance on your right leg while pulling your left knee into your chest. Grab your shin with both hands as if you were "hugging" your knee into your chest. Remain balanced by breathing in through your nose and out through your mouth in a calm and rhythmic fashion. Stay in that position for 20 seconds. Repeat on the opposite side for 20 seconds. You are welcome to repeat another set of 20 seconds per side if you were challenged or really enjoyed the exercise.

Your Fitness Footnote for today is to BREATHE!

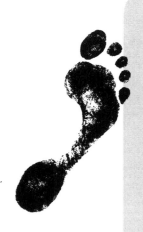

Breathing is one of the most basic things we do every day, however, it is amazing how little we know or understand about how the proper breathing technique can INSTANTLY change your life! Without breath we die, but with the proper breath we can not only live but do so in a clear, balanced and more peaceful place. The proper technique to increase your vitality through breathing is to focus on your breath. When you focus on your breathing, you allow the calming oxygen that enters your body each time you inhale to oxygenate and energize your blood and feed every muscle in your body. Proper breathing also increases your mental awareness, clarity and well-being. By breathing in deeply through your nose and exhaling forcefully out of your mouth you create a powerful rhythm that will increase your power and output capacity by 8 to 10%. That means you run longer, hit harder, and remain mentally focused by simply breathing properly. Your new healthy habit will benefit greatly if you focus on your BREATHING!

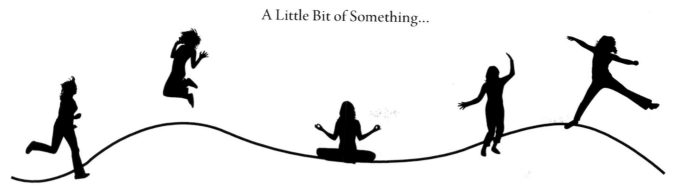

Journal the Journey

We all have to breathe to live. We all have to do it, but few of us do it with the proper technique that maximizes the air we breathe and minimize the stress we receive. To really reap the full benefit of proper breathing, let's learn a quick breathing exercise. Sit in a comfortable position and relax but don't slouch (neck straight, chest up, shoulders down and relaxed and back flat). Flair your nostrils as you pull in air through your nose (inhale for four sec) hold your breath for five seconds and blow out the carbon dioxide (exhale for four seconds). Continue this rhythmic breathing for three minutes and then proceed with your day. This breathing exercise also functions as an opportunity to meditate, pray, or simply quiet your mind. Repeat as often as you need to throughout your day and utilize this technique, in through the nose and out of the mouth, to help you increase your stamina whenever you exert energy.

37

DAy
15

"Positive thinking is expecting, talking, believing and visualizing what you want to achieve. It is seeing what you want as an accomplished fact."
~ Unknown

Today's little bit of something is doing "regular" push-ups for 45 seconds. A regular push-up means that your hands and toes are supporting you vs. the modified push up, where your knees are on the floor. It will be very important to breath properly to maximize the exercise. Breathe in deeply through your nose as you lower your body six inches off the ground and exhale out your mouth forcefully as you push back up into your starting position. Remember to push your elbows back not out to the side when you lower your body and keep your core tight (squeezing your tummy) and back flat throughout the exercise. Do as many "regular" push-ups as you can in 45 seconds. You are always encouraged to do more if you're able to and if you can't do one of the regular push-ups, then begin with modified push-ups, still watching your posture.

Your Fitness Footnote for today is to be POSITIVE!

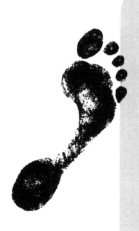

We are all blessed with an amazing gift often referred to as free will. It allows us to choose how we react to circumstances of life. With this free will we can determine our attitude, our perspective and ultimately our life. We can take a negative, pessimistic and fear-based approach that leads to a lack of power, failure and an unfulfilled life or we can embrace a positive approach that will lead to a powerful, successful and fulfilled life. The choice seems obvious when we look at it that way. Negative energy creates negative vibrations that repel the positive forces in nature. A bad attitude only gets worse because it is attracting more of the same negative energy being released. A positively charged person will release positive energy and vibrations that radiate out into the world and attract more positive energy back to the source. A positive attitude and outlook generates more creativity, balance, collaboration and success. Remain positive as you develop your new healthy habit in 30 days and share your "good vibrations."

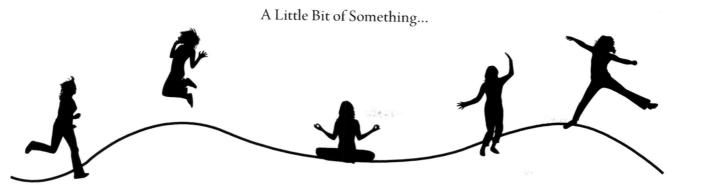

Journal the Journey

Being positive is probably one of the most powerful things we can actually CHOOSE to be! We don't need money, fame, a house, a degree, a car or anything at all to be positive! We simply have to decide, no matter what, that we will remain positive through whatever circumstances we are faced with! Today I want you to remain positive all day by employing a powerful strategy for change. Find a rubber-band and wear it as your "positivity reminder." Every time you feel a negative emotion or feeling begin to overwhelm you, SNAP OUT OF IT by snapping the rubber-band to stop your negative thought in its tracks. The slight discomfort from the pop will immediately refocus you on your positive outlook. Wear your "positivity reminder" as long as you need to in order to create your new healthy habit!

39

DAY 16

"If you have only one smile in you, give it to the people you love. Don't be surly at home, then go out in the street and start grinning 'Good morning' at total strangers."

~ Maya Angelou

Your little bit of something for today is to do "Get -Ups" from your back for 45 seconds. To do this exercise, start from a standing position and lie all the way down on your back with your arms stretched over your head. From that position, use your core strength (with no help from your elbows or hands) to sit upright, then you can use your hands to push yourself back onto your feet into a full standing position. I call this move "The Get-Up" or "Super Sit-Up." Getting up and down from the ground is a very functional exercise and will increase your blood flow, balance and athleticism. You are only required to do as many as you can in 30 seconds, but you are welcome to do another 45 second round of "Super Sit-Ups" if you are able.

Your fitness footnote for today is to show your LOVE!

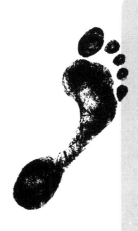

A happy, healthy life is built upon a foundation of love. Love drives just about every other emotion we feel. Love can make us happy or sad; it can make us good or bad, it can make us healthy or sick. It can even make us poor or rich. Love goes beyond the romanticized image that Hollywood and Madison Ave have so carefully crafted to sell movies, music and anything they can market. Love is the essence of our present, past and future! Love must begin with yourself in order for you to honestly love anyone else; and authentic love for yourself starts with your health! The greatest gift we have been endowed with is the gift of life itself... so what better way to demonstrate your love for yourself and your Creator than to take the very best care of your temple! By loving yourself enough to minimize stress, move responsibly as well as eat healthy and nutritious food, you will have the energy and capacity to love those in your family, your community and humanity in a more authentic and sincere way. Showing your love will help create your new healthy habit in 30 days!

40

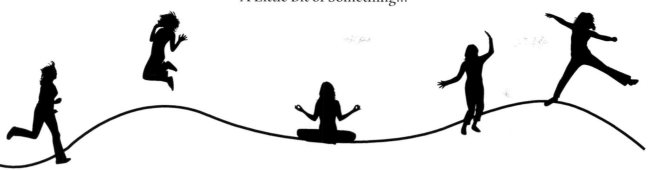

Journal the Journey

LOVE is a powerful emotion indeed! The best way to show your love for anything or anybody is to DO more to demonstrate as opposed to just articulate your appreciation. Love starts with yourself! Today I want you to recall and write down three reasons why you love YOURSELF. We often believe that if we demonstrate love for ourselves, we are vain, self-centered, or selfish, but a healthy love and respect for yourself is essential if you are to have the capacity to love and respect anyone else. Write down what it is about you that makes you the unique, valuable, and worthy individual you are and then DO something to help build, maintain or improve on an area that will make you love yourself even more. Love you some you today!

41

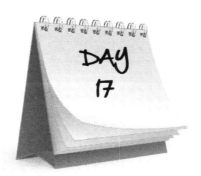

DAY
17

"To be nobody but myself-in a world which is doing its best, night and day, to make me somebody else-means to fight the hardest battle any human can fight, and never stop fighting."
~ E.E. Cummings

Your little bit of something for today is to do "Zombie Walks" for 30 seconds. This exercise is designed to work your core as well as stretch and tone your hips and thighs. To do the Zombie Walk, stand tall (chest up shoulders down and back) and extend both arms out in front like a zombie. Next, swing your right leg (don't bend your knee) up toward your extended right hand and then return to your starting position. Repeat the same move with your left leg. Keep alternating your legs or "walking" in place for 30 full seconds. Not only will this move improve your flexibility and balance, but it will also provide a good cardio workout if you swing your legs rapidly enough. You are encouraged to do two rounds of Zombie Walks if you are up to it but only one round is required.

Your Fitness Footnote for today is to Keep it REAL!

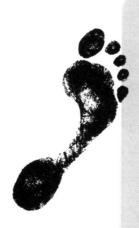

We live in a world full of delusion that has been created to keep us distracted and confused. A distracted and confused individual is unable to assess and ultimately solve the major issues causing harm, hurt or discomfort. The delusional images of beauty, success, health and happiness we are force-fed through "popular culture" creates an unrealistic standard that only serves to separate us from our own natural beauty and rugged individualism. For instance, the "lose weight fast" myth only distracts us from the real work of being committed to health.

Keeping it real is the best remedy for delusional or distracted thinking. It is simply seeing the situation for what it is and not what you've been told or sold. Keeping it real is being proactive instead of reactive.

Always operate from a place of authenticity. Be your natural self...eat natural food...breath natural air...and experience natural healing and holistic exercise. Keeping it REAL will ensure you create your new healthy habit in 30 days!

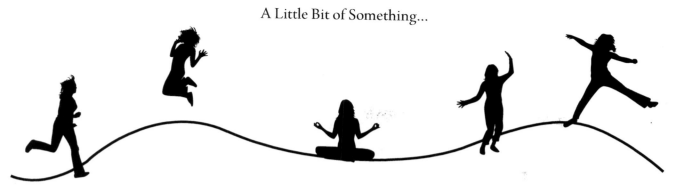

Journal the Journey

Our world is full of distractions! Things that hijack our focus and attention from what we really need to be focused on only serve to keep us stuck in neutral and never getting in the right "gear" of life. When you are overwhelmed with external "programming" from the music, film, television and social media outlets it becomes increasingly more difficult to originate your own authentic thoughts and opinions regarding your health, wealth, and society and your place in it. Today recall and write down three things that distract you from creating the life you desire and deserve... keep it real! Once you've identified your distractions, write three things you will do to minimize and reduce them...once again... keep it real! Operating from a place of authenticity, as opposed to a distracted mind, will allow you to shift into high gear and achieve the life you desire and deserve.

*"We are all manufacturers — some make a way,
others make progress, still others make excuses."*
~ Author Unknown

Today's little bit of something is to perform a lunge. The lunge is the best all-around exercise you can do to build muscle and balance in your lower body. The lunge activates and stimulates the muscles in your thighs, butt, hips and core all at the same time! Here is how it's done: start by standing straight and tall then take a big step forward with your right leg and plant your right foot into the ground. Bend your back knee (until it is just above the ground) and keep your chest up and back flat as you sink down into a lowered lunge position. Be sure your knee has not jutted out past the toes, but is in-line with the ankle. Hold for two seconds and then push off your right heel to return to your standing position. Repeat the exact same thing with the left leg. Keep alternating from right to left for 40 seconds. You are encouraged, as always, to do as many rounds as you can.

Your Fitness Footnote for today is to REDUCE THE EXCUSES!

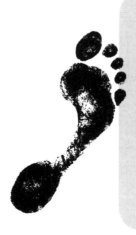

One of the best ways to sabotage yourself is to assign blame for your failures to anything or anybody but yourself. You relinquish your power to change when you confess you "don't have"...... whether you "don't have" enough time, talent, money, education or whatever excuses that keep you stuck where you don't want to be. When you change your perspective and stop making excuses, you will go from the "don't have" mindset to the "be" reality. The "be" reality is the mindset that believes that you can "be" smarter, "be" more disciplined, "be" tougher, "be" more committed to change and "be" more successful in everything you do! You must reduce the excuses in order to maximize your new healthy habit in 30 days and "be" healthier and happier for the rest of your life!

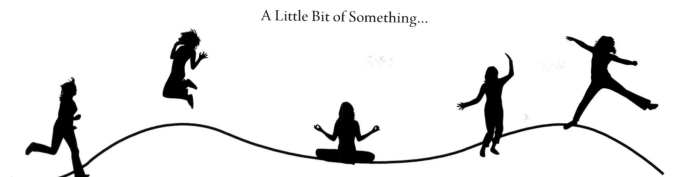

Journal the Journey

We justify our failed attempts by using excuses to soften the impact of falling short. In order to truly learn how to "fail forward" and maximize the real benefits of a failed attempt; take ownership of the outcome and learn exactly what you need to do (or not do) on your next attempt. Lamenting and creating excuses only serves to weaken your confidence, steal your focus, and undermine your chances for success. Today I want you to recall and write down the three excuses you use most often when it comes to your health and fitness. It could be your lack of time (a major excuse for many), your lack of knowledge, your lack of money, or your lack of motivation that sabotage your best efforts to start and maintain your new healthy habit. Whatever your excuses are, write them down now. Once you have recalled and written each excuse, write the word LIE in bold print next to your excuses! Remind yourself that the excuse is a lie you have been repeatedly telling and training your mind to believe! The LIE ends right now! Today you reduce the excuse and increase your awareness to create the body and mind you desire and deserve.

45

"You can map out a fight plan or a life plan, but when the action starts, it may not go the way you planned, and you're down to your reflexes - that means your [preparation:]. That's where your roadwork shows. If you cheated on that in the dark of the morning, well, you're going to get found out now, under the bright lights."
~ Smoking Joe Frazier

Your little bit of something for today is to imagine you are a world class boxer and shadow box. If you have never heard the term "shadow box," it simply means to throw punches at an imaginary opponent and that is exactly what you will be doing. To begin, if you are right handed, start in a staggered standing position with your right leg back and left leg forward (reverse if your left handed) and "put your dukes up"… raise your left fist in front of your nose and your right fist slightly behind it with your elbows tucked by your rib cages. Start the session by taking your left fist and punching across your body (rotating your shoulders and hips in the direction of the punch) and quickly return to your starting position. Count out 20 punches with your left hand (jab). After you complete your jabs, repeat the same process with the right fist.

Your Fitness Footnote for today is to FIGHT FOR YOUR FITNESS!

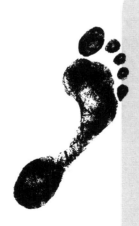

Life is a worthy opponent. Sometimes it can seem like waves of troubles are constantly crashing down upon you. As soon as you seem to get one situation together, another one comes crashing down, knocking you off balance and disorienting your position. After repeated times getting knocked to your knees, you may feel like you are unable to defend yourself; and so you throw in the towel. Your fitness struggle may seem like a similar battle. With processed food everywhere, a lack of time and stressful situations constantly coming your way, you may feel like the waves of life are crashing down on every attempt you make at getting fit and healthy. You may feel like you are either too far gone or just not able to stay consistent to a wellness program. Either way, you may have thrown in the towel and decided to simply hope for the best when it comes your health and wellness. You cannot win if you don't show up for the fight!

If you forfeit the fight for your fitness by not eating intelligently, moving responsibly and educating yourself accordingly, you are not just quitting on yourself but you are quitting on all the people who rely on you in your family, in your profession and in humanity! Change your perspective, your strategy or your team. Do whatever you need to do to stay in the fight! You must fight for your fitness like your life depends on it... because it actually does! Deciding to fight for your fitness will help you achieve your new healthy habit in 30 Days.

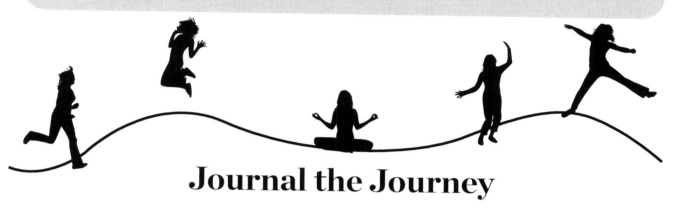

Journal the Journey

Sometimes life can feel like a bully! Life can appear to push us around and keep us defensive if we allow it. But like with most bullies, if you show no fear and stand your ground, you can turn the tables and regain your power. Life is not dictated by your conditions as much as it is by your decisions! No matter what condition you may currently be in physically, financially or mentally, you can change it with the decision to do what you need to do to FIGHT for your FUTURE! Today I want you to write down three things regarding your health and wellness worth fighting for such as more exercise, healthier meals, time to meditate/pray, family time, time outside, better stress management, etc.

47

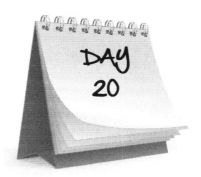

DAY 20

"The doctor of the future will give no medicines, but will interest his patients in the care of the human frame, in diet, and in the causes and prevention of disease."
~ *Thomas Edison*

Your little bit of something for today is to run in place for 30 seconds. This simple move can be done anywhere and really gets your heart and lungs beating in a very short period of time. To maximize this exercise keep your back flat and chest up as you drive your knees up and down while pumping your relaxed fist from your hips to your lips and breathing rhythmically in through your nose out your mouth. Try to remain on your toes throughout the exercise (to maximize calf engagement) and land gently as you impact the ground to prevent jarring your joints and putting unnecessary pressure on your body. As always, you're encouraged to do as many 30 second rounds as your able.

Your fitness footnote is to be PROACTIVE!

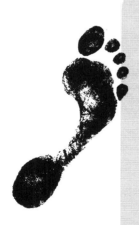

Much too often we allow the ups and downs of life to dictate our reality. We are blown about, like leaves in the wind, because we would rather "play it safe" and allow life to happen to us as opposed to "play it fearless" and effect what happens in our lives. We often live life reacting to the circumstances and situations life throws at us as opposed to proactively dictating and directing the course we ultimately would have our lives take. Instead of engaging in preventive measures, like eating better, exercising more, reducing stress and becoming healthier, we typically wait until we experience pain, discomfort or disease before we react to our unfortunate condition. Reacting often reduces our quality of life by forcing us to deal with issues that may have been prevented while incurring cost that could have been avoided. Through being proactive, you increase your quality of life by preventing injuries and illness; and controlling that which you can control. Be proactive in the pursuit of your new healthy habit and watch your health habit reward your efforts!

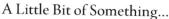

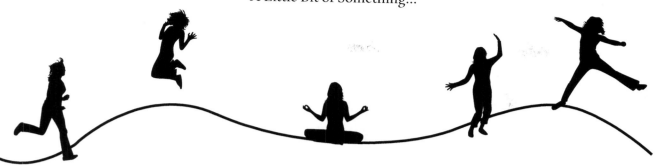

Journal the Journey

Many people live life simply on the surface. For some folks, having a popular personality is of paramount importance. They develop their presentation, wardrobe and style but oftentimes neglect the substance that would allow them to activate their ability to respond (responsibility) to any given situation. I call this type of person a personality driven individual. There are other people who live and operate beneath the surface. They have built principles and values into their personal foundation which give them the ability to respond (responsibility) to any circumstances and to proactively prevent many pitfalls from occurring in the first place. Today I want you to write down three core principles you live by (faith, honesty, loyalty, love, forgiveness, fairness, respect, authenticity, fearlessness, curiosity, etc.). Once you have done that, write down how those principles can help you be more proactive regarding your health and wellness. Use your principle power to proactively provide the platform for your new healthy habit.

49

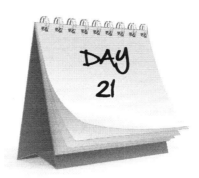

DAY 21

"At the center of your being you have the answer; you know who you are and you know what you want."

~ Lao Tzu

Your little bit of something for today is a very simple (but not easy) exercise that will really work your core (abs, oblique's, lower back) called "Six Inches." To perform this exercise, lay flat on your back. Brace your lower back by forming a diamond shape with both hands and placing that diamond comfortably in the small of your back. Once you are in position, simply lift both feet six inches off the floor and hold the position for five seconds. Repeat four more times, bringing your total time to 20 seconds. Don't forget to breathe in deeply through your nose and forcefully out of your mouth while you hold the position. As always, you are encouraged to do more if you are able to.

Your Fitness Footnote for today is to find your CENTER!

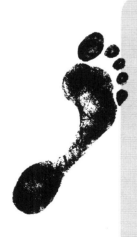

We are all motivated by many things in life. Family, spouse, career, money, children, church, social groups and whatever else all vie for our time and attention. We are connected with and concerned about so many people and "things" that we seldom stop to find our motivational or creative center. We may believe we are centered on our family and their happiness and protection, which is admirable. We may feel like we are centered on our career and the climb to the top of our profession. We may even believe we are centered on ourselves at times; our own need to experience the pleasure and variety life. But your center is your creative energy that resonates from the inside out, not from the outside in. Although you may deeply love and protect your family, appreciate and excel at your profession or worship and serve at your church, all those things are external and subject to change. Children grow up, jobs and professions phase in and out and churches change leaders, people and locations. What will never change are the principles and values that make up your character and core. Although kids grow up and spouses grow old, the fundamental love, loyalty and respect that you have as principles of life will never change.

Jobs and professions may come and go, but your work ethic, honesty, and knowledge will remain constant. Churches may change pastors or places, but your faith, conviction and gratitude will never waiver if it is a principle core value at the center of your life. Take time to identify your core values and creative center which you resonate to the world. Knowing your center will tremendously assist you in creating your new healthy habit in 30 days.

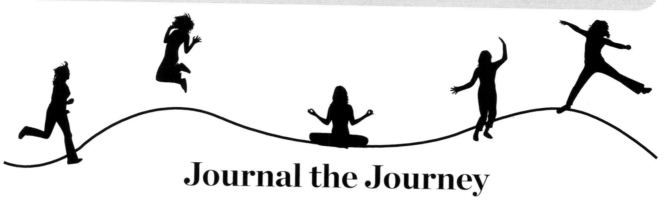

Journal the Journey

Life is constantly changing, but it is important for us to always know where our emotional center is located. Like a surfer riding the wave of his life, we must remain balanced, focused and fearless. No matter how far to the right or left life takes us; we must always find our way back to the middle or our emotional center. Today I want you to recall and write down three character traits that someone else might associate with you (honest, loyal, hardworking, ethical, etc.). Then write down three character traits that you would associate with yourself... be honest! Examine your list carefully because it is a very good chance that your list is an inventory of your emotional core, the values you consider important enough to live by.

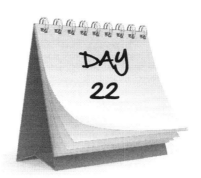

"Strong minds discuss ideas, average minds discuss events, weak minds discuss people."
~Socrates

Your little bit of something for today is to eat three servings of vegetables. You can blend, juice or cook your veggies, but you have to consume three servings today. Absolutely everything we need to live a healthy, whole life is given to us by our creator. The water rains down naturally from the sky, the fruits and vegetables grow naturally from the earth, and your exercise will happen naturally if you simply go out into nature and play. As sure as the sun shines to help elevate your mood, your body will respond when you eat natural food. As usual, you are encouraged to continue to eat as much naturally grown and prepared food every day to help maximize weight loss and health restoration.

Your Fitness Footnote for today is to direct your DISCUSSION!

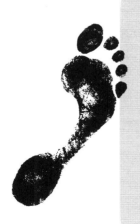

People love to talk! We love to talk about our favorite show, our favorite restaurants and our favorite entertainer! But is this discussion developing or destroying your mental and physical health and wellness? Are you talking about techniques and strategies that will actually help you accomplish your goals or are you just complaining about the things you don't have or can't do? Are you studying and discussing people that could enlighten and empower you or are you idolizing and gossiping about people who could care less about you? Are you speaking courage, abundance and life in your daily discussion or fear, lack and death? Words are extremely powerful, so direct the discussions you have to develop your awareness and education as often as you can to insure you maximize your new healthy habit in 30 days.

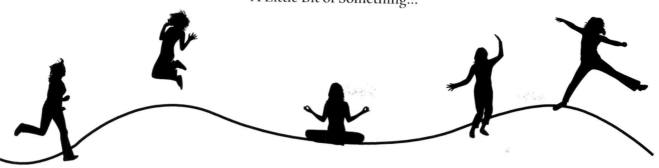

Journal the Journey

If you were born with two eyes, two ears and one mouth, the creator must have designed you to listen and observe twice as much as you speak! This old saying is as full of wisdom today as it was when it was first uttered. We live in a world where there is constant chatter. People continually talk about "stuff" consumes our thought process, distracts our decision making and stagnates our intentions. When we get caught up in the currents of the mainstream conversations about people, places, and things, we tend to lose focus on what's truly essential for our evolution. Today, listen to the conversations around you with a renewed focus and decipher what is useful and what is just "noise," then write two columns, one which lists the useful things you heard and one which outlines the noise. When you are aware of the noise, you can turn the volume on that down and increase the volume on the things that will build the life you desire and deserve!

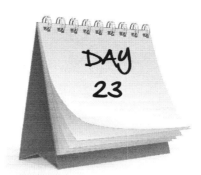

"Without education, you're not going anywhere in this world."
~Malcolm X

Your little bit of something for today is to exercise good posture all day. Rounded backs and hunched over shoulders put an extra strain on your neck and lower back as well your diaphragm and lungs. Your oxygen flow is compromised, so you don't think as clearly, function as effectively, or react as quickly to stimuli. Good posture is simply sitting straight, with your back flat, chest up and shoulders (relaxed) down and back. This proper position will align your spine and relieve your diaphragm. Additionally, it will decrease pressure on your lower back and increase your positive blood flow. You are encouraged to exercise good posture all day today and each day going forward. Be conscious of your posture!

Your Fitness Footnote for today is to EDUCATE YOURSELF!

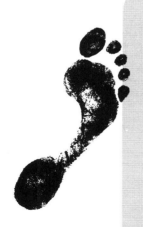

Many of us erroneously believe that real education ends the day we graduate from high school or college. The reality is that education truly begins the moment we leave the comfortable confines of our "formal" education system. School was implemented to give students a well-rounded, liberal education on life in general, but the details and real decisions of life are typically learned as we live. Life has definitely taught us that our health and wellness is essential to the success of everything else in life. If you are sick, you spend your time, energy and money on trying to get healthy again. A quality fitness and health education can literally mean the difference between life and death in our current society. Ignorance, when it comes to nutrition and exercise, cause people to live sicker and die younger. Continue to edify your education by being curious about what you eat, how you move and the ways you relax and "decompress" the stresses of life. Continuing your education will empower your new healthy habit in 30 days!

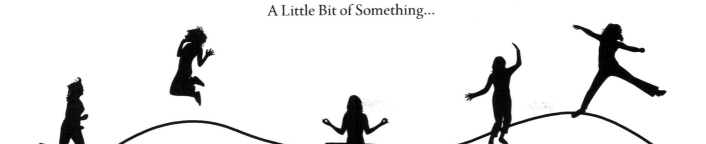

Journal the Journey

Education is the key that opens the door to your future. The process of evolution begins the moment we empower ourselves with new, relevant and transformational information and education. We live in the most amazing time in history regarding our access to information. In our pockets lie the gateway to the entire scope of human knowledge, organized, categorized and easily accessed. The internet does not discriminate, intimidate or refuse access to anyone with a connection and the curiosity to want to know more. Today, I want you to explore your curiosity and research three topics that will increase your pool of knowledge. Write down the three topics you are going to explore and highlight or bullet point some of the more interesting facts you read. Most people operate with a shallow pool of information (limited to only what's necessary to get by) but enlightened people operate with deep wells of information and education (limited only by their curiosity). Educate yourself today!

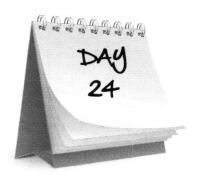

"The big picture can't be seen by those without vision"
~Tony Robbins

Your little bit of something for today is to 5 Burpees. What in the world is a Burpee? you ask. The Burpee happens to be one of the best full body exercises you can do. It combines muscle building, fat burning and cardio conditioning into one effective exercise. To do a Burpee, start from a standing position, then squat down (legs open wider than you shoulders) and place both hands on the ground. From here, explosively kick both feet straight back (you'll end up in a push up position). To finish, bring both feet back under your body in a squat position (feet should be wider than your hands) then hop back up into your starting position. That's one repetition. Try to do 5 Burpees if you can and, as always, you're encouraged to do as many as you're able to do if 5 is not enough of a challenge.

Your fitness footnote for today is to keep your eye on the BIG PICTURE!

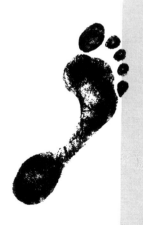

Life has a great way of forcing us to focus on the immediate "fires" we daily encounter and forfeit the long term vision needed to prevent future "fires" from cropping up and consuming everything. For example, busy parents are consistently seeking ways to juggle hectic schedules and feed their families an affordable, filling meal before bed. To solve the immediate problem, stressed parents may buy highly processed, pre-made microwave meals or stop by the local fast food joint to pick-up the latest "meal deal" for dinner. The immediate problem may be solved, but the solution has created another, more dangerous problem ahead. The kids go to bed full, but the food they ate may cause them to be overweight and unhealthy. We saw the snapshot, and not the big picture! When we see the Big Picture as opposed to just the snapshot, we are able to start with the end in mind and work backward. If the Big Picture idea is to have our kids grow up to be fit, healthy adults, then we must invest the time, resources and discipline needed right now to insure that will be their future reality. The same idea applies to every facet of your life.

By knowing what you want your Big Picture to look like, you're able to manage the "snapshots" of life so they create the Big Picture you envision! Keeping your Big Picture in mind will help you maximize your new healthy habit.

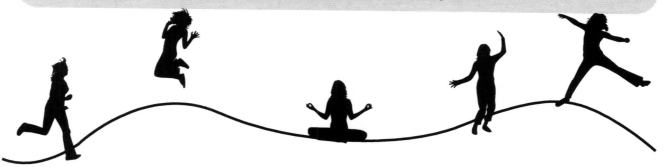

Journal the Journey

How do you want your life to look 1, 2 or 3 years from now? Do you have a vision or "big picture" of what you want for yourself and your family? If you don't, or if you do and it's not clear enough, then today is for you! I want you to imagine what the end of your life will look like, and write your own epithet. What will people remember you for? What did you stand for, what did you fall for? Did you put money over people or people over money? Were you honest and intelligent in your business and financial dealings? Were you healthy and stress free? Imagine what you want your life to look like later so you can begin to paint the picture right now with your current actions and attitudes.

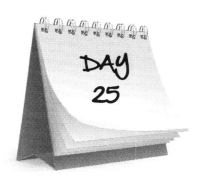

"As a general rule, teachers teach more by what they are than by what they say."
~ Anonymous

Your little bit of something for today is calf raises. To do this move, simply stand tall and raise yourself onto your tip toes, hold for five seconds, then drop your heels back down. Repeat that basic move nine more times for a total of 10 repetitions. You are encouraged to do more if you are up to it.

Your Fitness Footnote for today is to TEACH others how to be healthy!

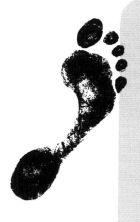

Our society is sick on so many levels. Obesity and disease are certainly making folks sick, but our mental health and well-being, along with our moral and spiritual center, is also being attacked. In order to change our current reality, we need those who have survived great challenges to teach and inspire the struggling masses how to overcome as well. The people closest to the conflict are always the real experts. Therefore, if you have learned a successful way to control your weight and remain healthy, teach it! If you have learned a way to successfully control stress, teach it! As you learn these new exercises and mental strategies, share if you care and each one teach one so we can build a healthy community. Teaching will be a very important part of developing and sharing your new healthy habit in 30 days!

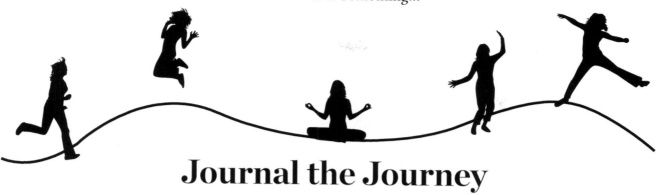

Journal the Journey

Teaching is essential to learning and learning is essential to living the life you desire and deserve. What are you teaching the people around you? Are they learning what to do or are they learning what not to do from you? We are all teachers in some capacity and when we are aware of the power we possess to influence and instill ideas into those we encounter, we will develop a respect for our power and use it wisely. Today teach three people something valuable that you know. It can be as simple as teaching someone how to play chess, do a proper push up, or wash a car without leaving spots or as complicated as a new language. Teach whatever you know and watch your confidence grow today!

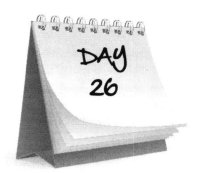

"Ultimately, the only power to which man should aspire is that which he exercises over himself."
~Elie Weisel

Your little bit of something for today is a light jog around your house. Sounds a little weird right... but the idea is to simply get your heart beating. Lightly jog into each room of your house (including your bathroom) and spend about 10 seconds in each room running in place. You are finished when you get back to where you started from. You are encouraged to go around the house as many times as you can, but only one is required.

Your Fitness Footnote for today is to harness your POWER!

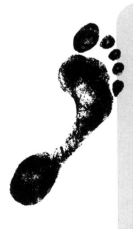

We are all endowed with super powers. We may not have the ability to fly, climb walls or lift buildings, but we can overcome monumental challenges, endure supernatural setbacks and bounce back from devastating defeats. We also have the power to change shape (through exercise and diet), forecast the future (by doing what you say you are going to do) and live forever (through the legacy we leave). Society has a tendency to suppress your super powers by manipulating you through the use of media and images. The media created image of beauty or fitness may not be your reality, so it chips away at the image you may hold of yourself, thereby weakening your powers slightly with each exposure. In order to harness your suppressed super powers, you have to no longer fear the opinion of other people! Your journey is your journey and the way other people feel about it should not concern you. The people who matter in your life won't mind your evolution, and the people who mind your evolution won't matter! Utilize your renewed powers to get healthier, wealthier and happier by activating your new healthy habit to change your reality!

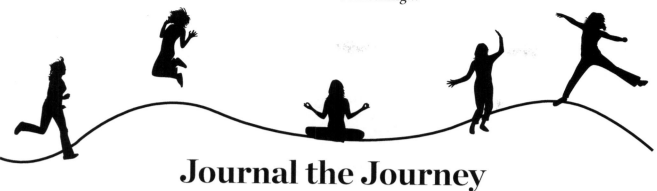

Journal the Journey

You are POWERFUL! Remember that! Life has a tendency to try to either steal your power or use it to build others people's dreams. The only way anything or anybody can take your power is if you give it away. Society is adept at distracting you from developing and harnessing your super powers in order to create the life you desire and deserve. Today I want you to recall and write down three talents you have that could qualify as a Superpower. It could be your supernatural patience, your supernatural gift of gab, or perhaps it could be your ability to relate and converse with anyone. Wherever you feel your power lies, write it down today and then utilize your power to effect a positive change for your life and the lives of your loved ones!

61

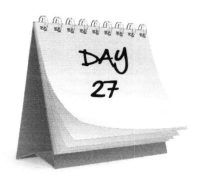

"When you are going through hell, keep on going. Never never never give up."
~ Winston Churchill

Your little bit of something for today is to jump rope for one minute. If you have a real jump rope handy, of course use it. If you don't have a jump rope, then simply imagine you do and mimic the moves as if you were holding a rope in your hands. Keep your chest up, shoulders relaxed and back flat as you bounce on your toes; breathe in through your nose and out through your mouth. 60 seconds will be sufficient but if you can jump longer, DO IT!

Your Fitness Footnote for today is to NEVER GIVE UP!

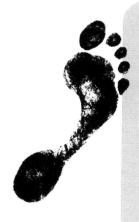

Sometimes we just get tired! We feel so overwhelmed by the trials and tribulations of the daily grind that we just want to say, "To hell with it" and throw in the towel. Although life may be a challenge, questioning our will and desire to change, we must remember to never give in, give out or give up on ourselves or our goals. The best way to insure you stay dedicated on your desire to get better and not quit is to plan your trip! If you plan your trip, you know where you are going; how long the trip should take and what resources you need to get there. Knowing what to expect helps you stay the course and endure setbacks because you can visualize the end result and know that problems don't and won't last forever. It's hard to give up when you can see the finish line! The hardest part of rolling a big rock is to start the rock rolling... once it's moving, momentum will take over and it becomes very hard to stop. Don't quit or give up on your new healthy habit, let it be a rolling rock, full of momentum that is hard to stop.

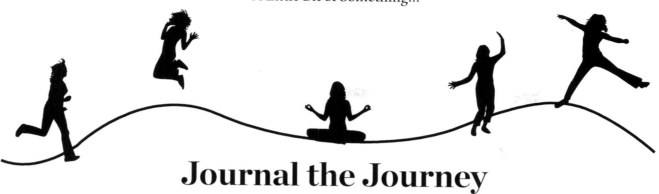

Journal the Journey

You must never quit! If your journey is arduous, quitting absolutely won't help it get any easier! As times get tough, the only choice a winner can make is to simply get tougher. Today I want you to recall and write down three obstacles tempting you to quit your struggle before you reach your desired results. Once written, I need you to then write the CONSEQUENCES of you quitting. Who will suffer the most if you quit? Will quitting improve your circumstances or make them worse? Will you feel better if you quit or push through and achieve your objectives? Decide to never give in, give out, or give up on YOU!

63

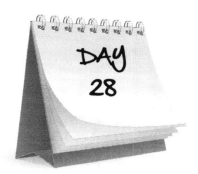

"Setting an example is not the main means of influencing others, it is the only means."
~Albert Einstein

Your little bit of something for today is to run hard outside for three minutes. Now I want you to really listen to your body during this brief but intense workout because it will challenge every muscle in your body. A hard run is basically sprinting at about 80 - 95% of your maximum speed. I suggest you stretch lightly before running and choose a soft surface (track, park, field, etc.) to run on. Keep your chest up, back flat and shoulders relaxed as you run. You can sprint for 10 seconds then rest for 20 seconds (or any similar variation) until you reach three minutes of total activity. If you are up for more, you are encouraged to do another two minutes of interval running.

Your Fitness Footnote for today is to be a good EXAMPLE for your family!

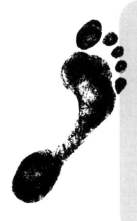

In order for the next generation to appreciate and cultivate a healthy, fit lifestyle, we must provide them with a positive example. We have to prioritize our exercise and focus on the food we buy; how we prepare it and how much we serve. We must be aware of the fact that every time we put something in our mind and mouth, we are either feeding or fighting disease! Show your family how to beat disease by demonstrating your dedication to exercise, proper nutrition and stress management through your daily action. Setting a good example will set you up for success in developing your new healthy habit in 30 days!

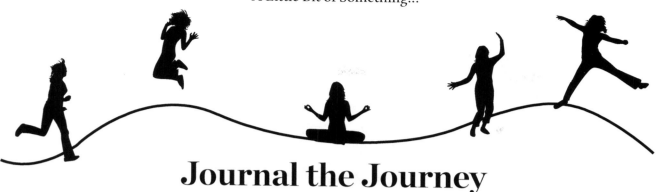

Journal the Journey

Our life is ultimately decided by our decisions, not our conditions. The way we respond to crisis, setbacks, or even success will influence not only our lives but it will also affect the lives of the people we influence. People remember what we do far longer than what we say so the example we set is of paramount importance. Today I want you to recall and write down the names of five people you influence and if your example is a positive, negative or neutral influence on them. If your example is anything other than positive, reexamine your motives and identify the ways you in which you can improve the way you influence and the example your creating through your actions.

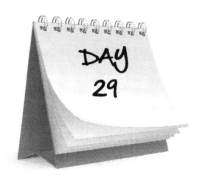

"Invest in your health because your health is the engine of your wealth."
~ Jay Jones, Fitness Minister

Your little bit of something for today is a simple (but not easy) full body exercise called the "Super Human Hop." This move will stimulate and develop your entire lower body as well as stretch and condition your upper body. To do this exercise, stand tall, then pull both your arms back as you push and lower your hips back and down into a squat position. From here, exhale forcefully as you swing your arms above your head and launch your body into the air! That's one rep. Now do as many as you can in 25 seconds. Try to launch and land in the same spot and lessen the impact on your knees by landing on your toes. As usual, you are encouraged to do more than the initial 25 seconds if you are up to it.

Your Fitness Footnote for today is to INVEST in your health!

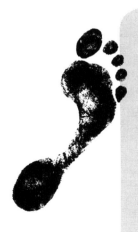

Americans spend a lot of money! Naturally, money is spent on the necessities of life (food, shelter, and clothing) but a lot of money is also spent on our habits, hobbies and family. Seldom do we invest in our health, the most important asset, until it begins to breakdown and cause discomfort and pain. For example, if you wait until you are sick to begin investing in your health, you are going to incur the cost of poor mental and physical health as well as the financial cost of doctors, hospitals, pharmaceutical companies and insurance providers that can actually bankrupt the average citizen. Alternatively, you can be proactive and invest in your health before you get sick by purchasing healthy food and hiring a fitness professional to help educate, inspire, and hold you accountable for your fitness. It is always cheaper to invest upfront as opposed to the back end. So please be encouraged to invest your resources wisely to maximize your new healthy habit in 30 days!

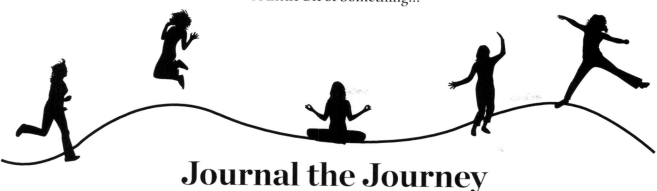

Journal the Journey

What are you investing in? Are you investing your resources on assets or liabilities? An asset adds value to you and a liability decreases your value. Our sick society loves to spend time, talents and money on liabilities when it comes to health and wellness. We enjoy our western diet and lifestyle comprised of the "treats" we have come to love! The burgers, pizzas, sodas, restaurants, bars, movies, internet and television all provide us with opportunities to invest our resources but will this investment feed or fight disease or build or destroy the life we desire and deserve? Where a person spends his/her treasure is what that individual values most, therefore your budget is your value statement. Today I want you to recall and write down the three investments you make the most on a daily basis. Are your investments paying you a positive return? If not, you may need to reallocate your resources to activities that will make you healthier, wealthier and happier!

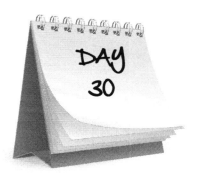

DAY 30

*"The more you praise and celebrate your life,
the more there is in life to celebrate."*
~Oprah Winfrey

Your little bit of something for today is to take a nap! We live in a sleep deprived society and in our quest to "make a dollar," we have forfeited some of the most fundamental facets of life, namely a good night's sleep. Rest is the body's natural rejuvenator, healer and decompression chamber. Rest may sound like an easy prescription, but we must find the time to fill it! My mother would always take a nap after work to prepare for the evening duties (cooking, cleaning and preparing my sister and I for another day) and that taught me the value of "finding" the time to rest, recover, and rejuvenate with a little sleep! I strongly recommend you take a quick nap to develop the energy you will need to maintain your new healthy habit!

Your Fitness Footnote for today is to CELEBRATE your victories!

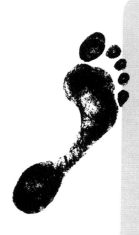

When we sacrifice to succeed and actually finish what we start, it is cause for a celebration! We typically celebrate birthdays, holidays and weddings along with the sporadic promotion and/or raise every now and then. But another way to approach celebration is to see it simply as the acknowledgement of having done something good; to recognize and rejoice in a job well done! We experience many small victories every day that go uncelebrated. When we celebrate, we encourage more of the same behavior so commemorate your big and small victories equally. Celebrate when you overcome your fatigue and fear and start that new workout group. Rejoice when you fight off the temptation to eat the whole bag and settle for a napkin full. Cheer when you don't allow anyone to steal your joy and peace because you OWN that! Finally, celebrate your new healthy habit of doing at least a little bit of something EVERYDAY to improve your mental, physical and Spiritual fitness! Now go forth and TEACH what you have LEARNED, superstar!

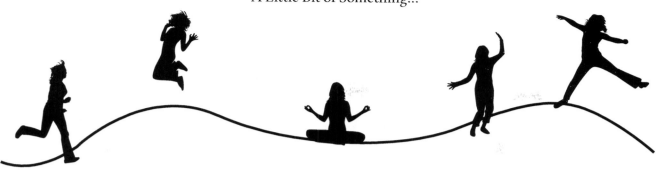

Journal the Journey

Congratulations! I am so proud of you for not giving in, giving out, or giving up on yourself and finishing this workbook! You have demonstrated your desire to learn the habit creation strategies in this book by being diligent, dedicated and disciplined. It's time to CELEBRATE! Today I want you to recall and write down three ways your new healthy habit of doing a little bit of something, as opposed to a whole lot of nothing, everyday is going to improve your life! I also want to celebrate with you personally by offering a live one-on-one training session via Skype to you absolutely free! It is my token of appreciation to you for allowing me to be of service and for you "doing what you said you were going to do" and finishing! I am proud of you on so many levels and cannot wait to meet you! You can reach me through the website *A Little Bit of Something.Today*. Stay focused, fearless and faithful and watch your new health habit bud, blossom and bear fruit in your life! God Bless you!

More
Journal the Journey
Pages

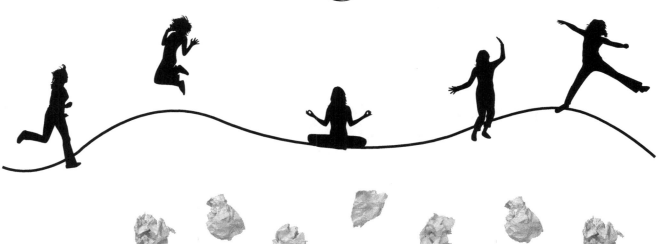

Continued from page _____

Continued from page _____

Continued from page _____

Continued from page _____

Continued from page _____

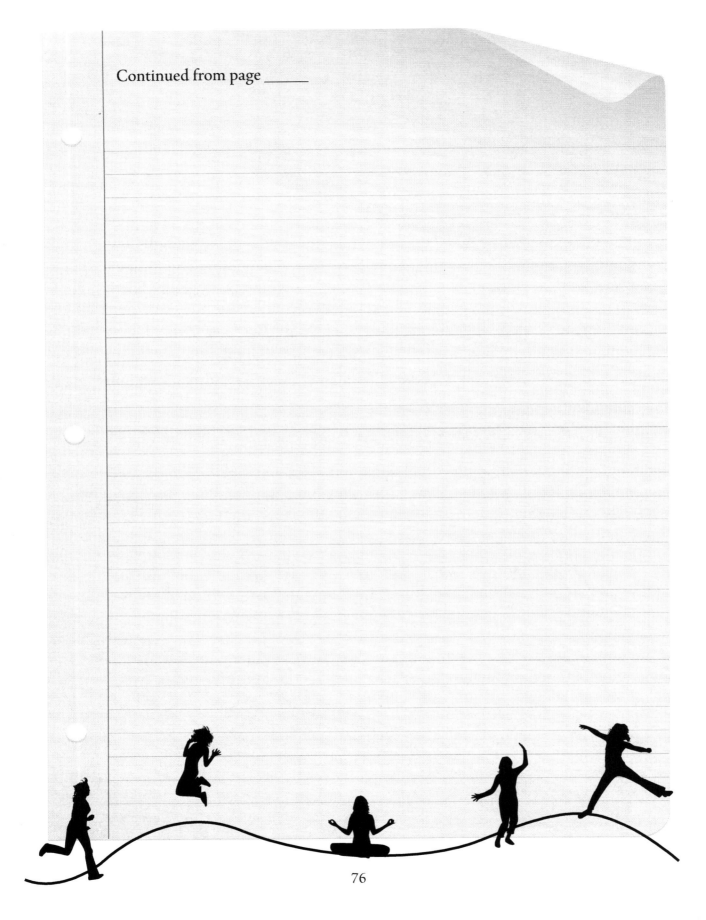

Continued from page _____

Continued from page _____

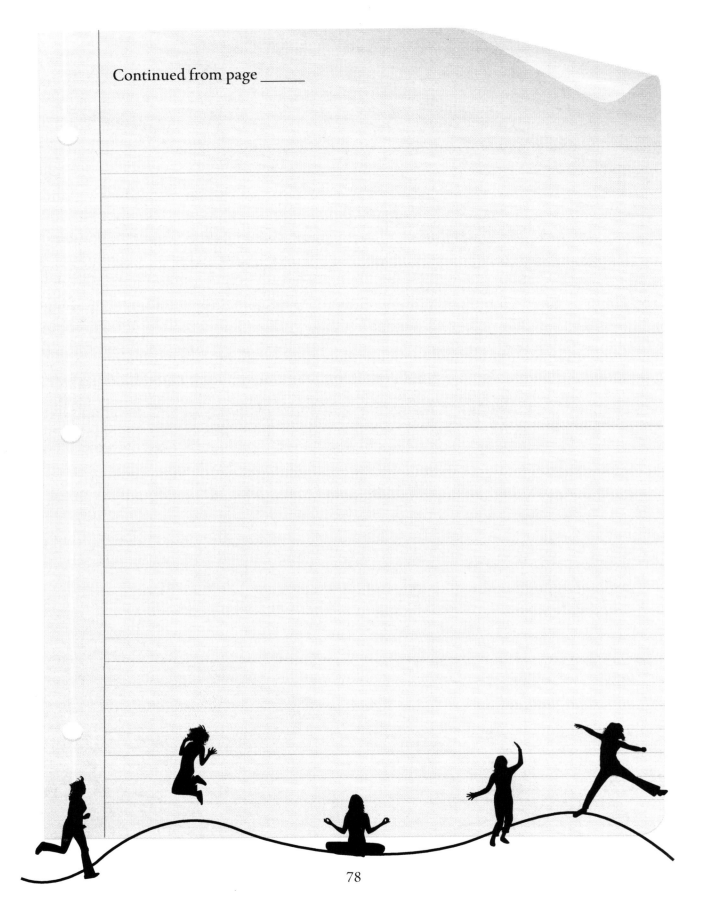

Continued from page _____

Continued from page _____

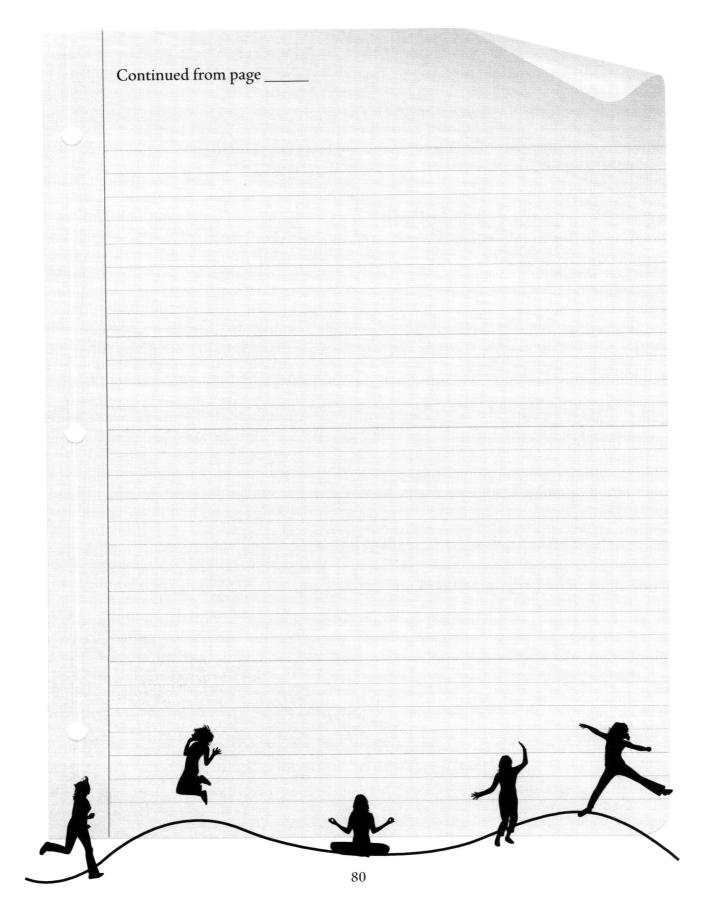

Continued from page _____

Continued from page _____

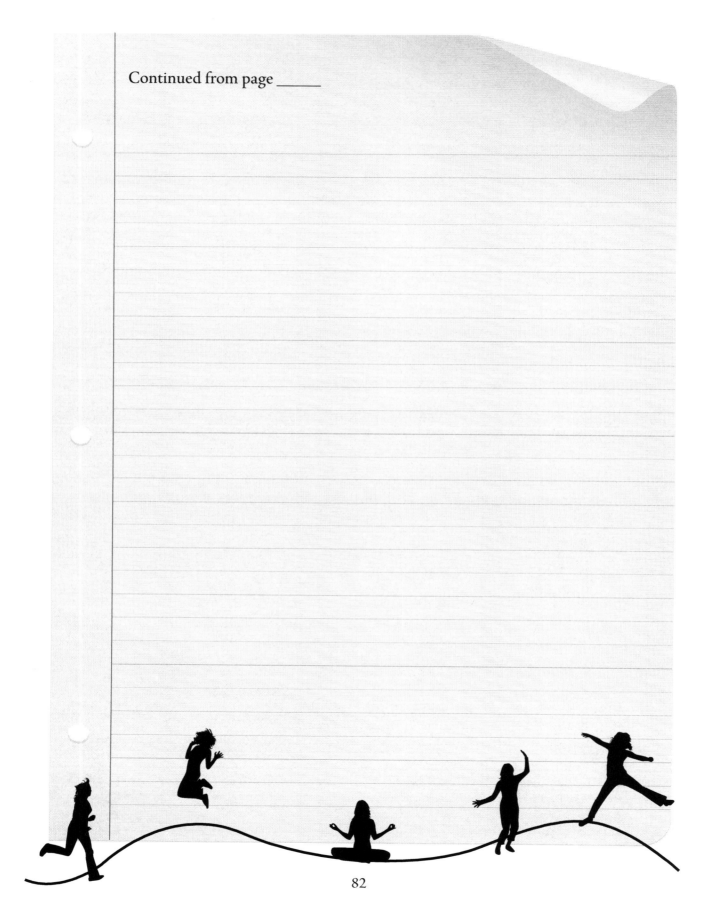

Continued from page _____

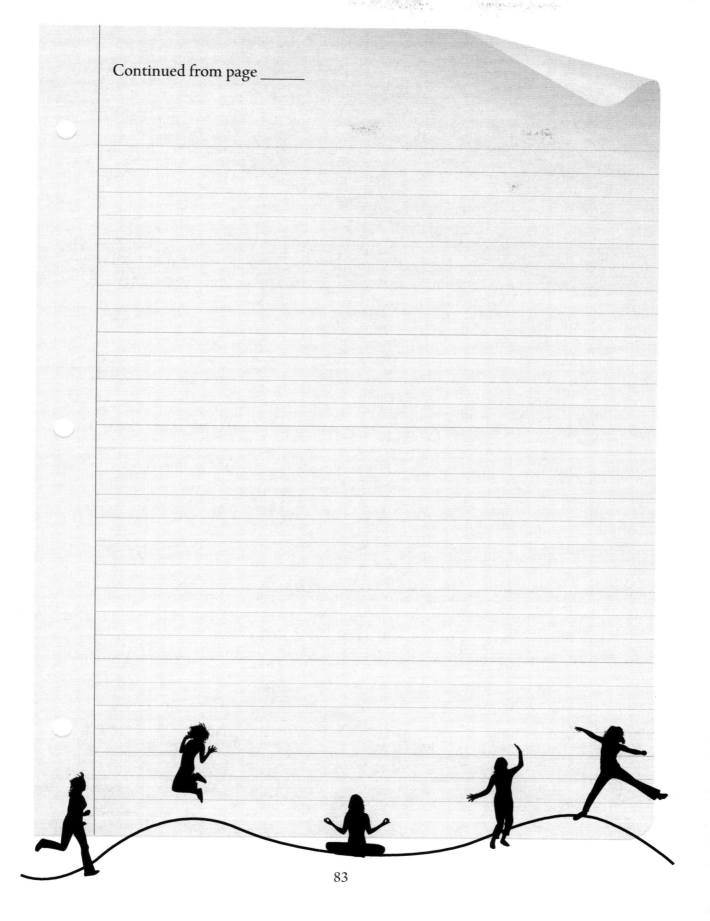

Continued from page _____

Continued from page _____

Continued from page _____

Continued from page _____

Continued from page _____

Continued from page _____

Continued from page _____

Continued from page _____

Continued from page _____

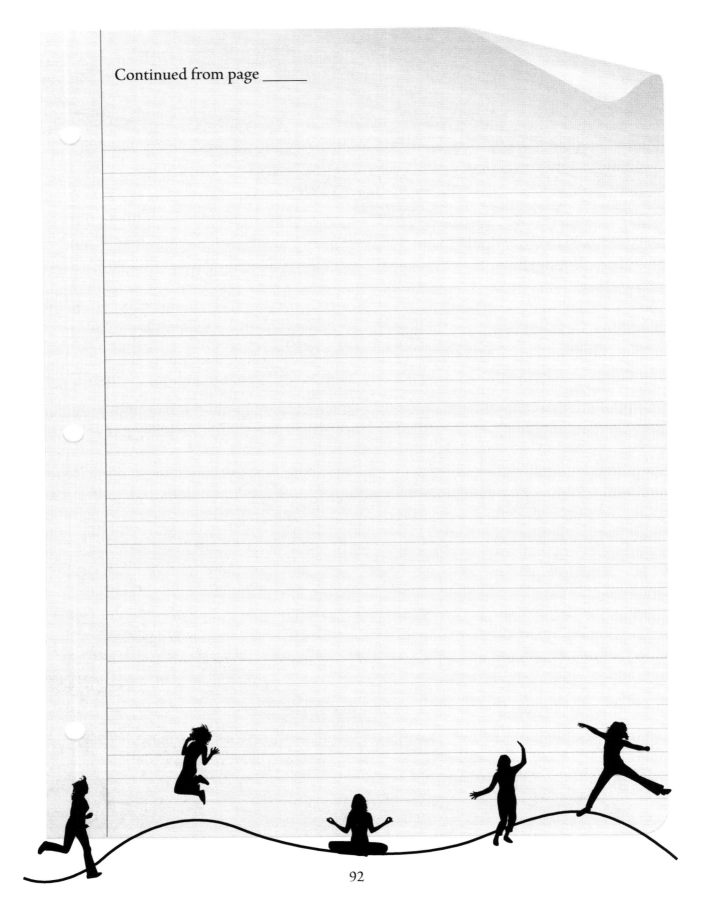

Continued from page _____

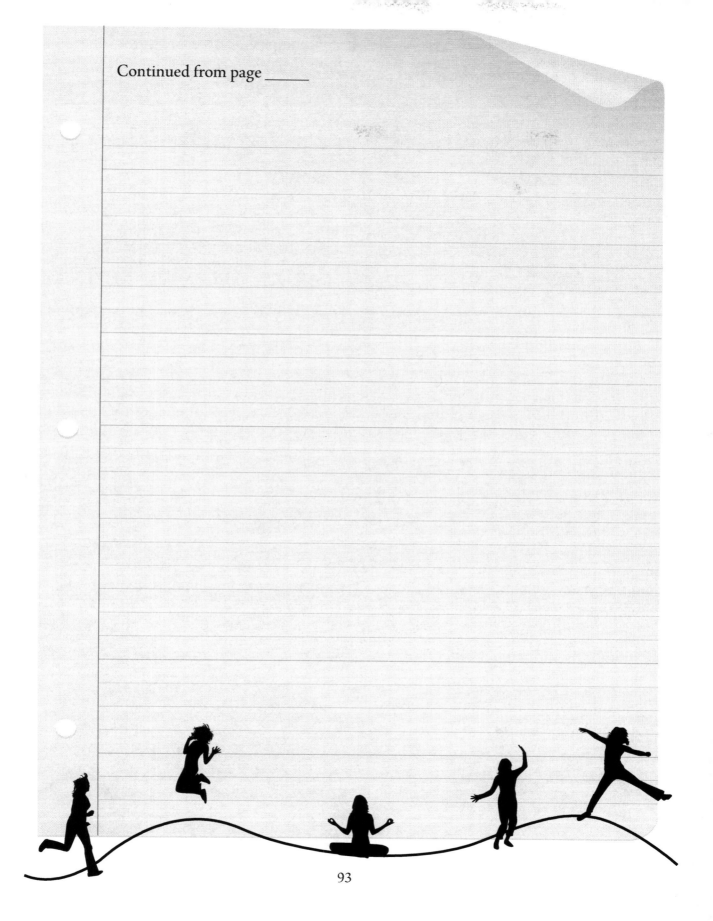

Continued from page _____

Continued from page _____

Continued from page _____

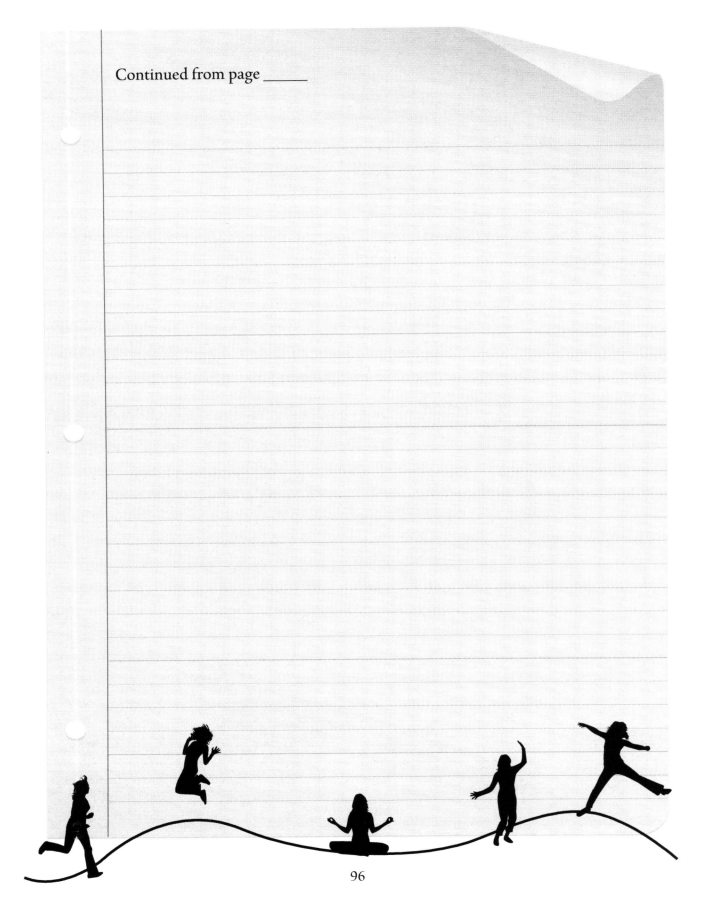

Continued from page _____

Continued from page _____

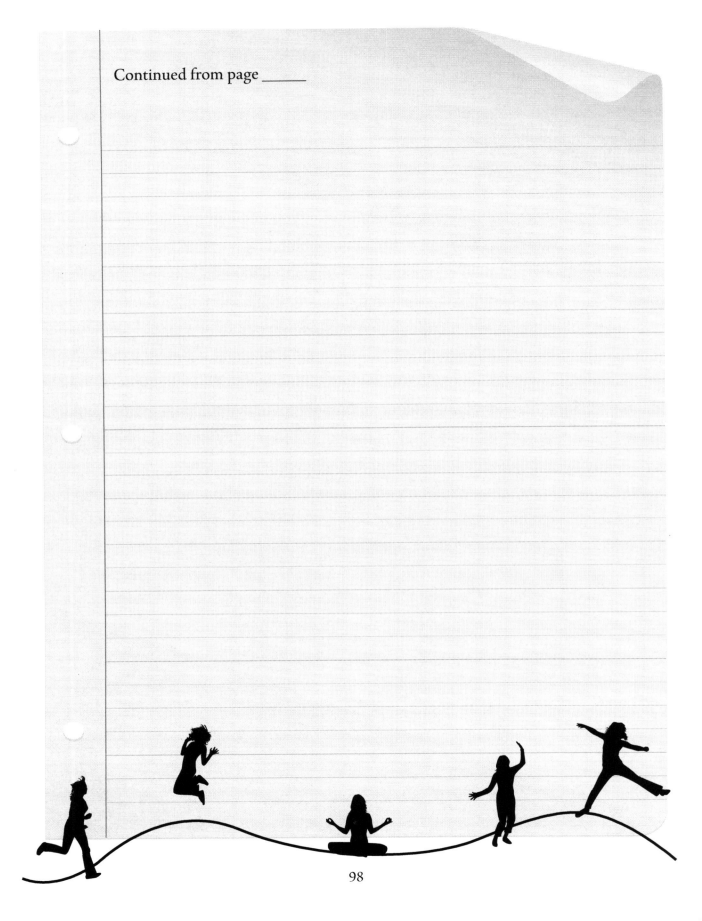

Continued from page _____

Continued from page _____

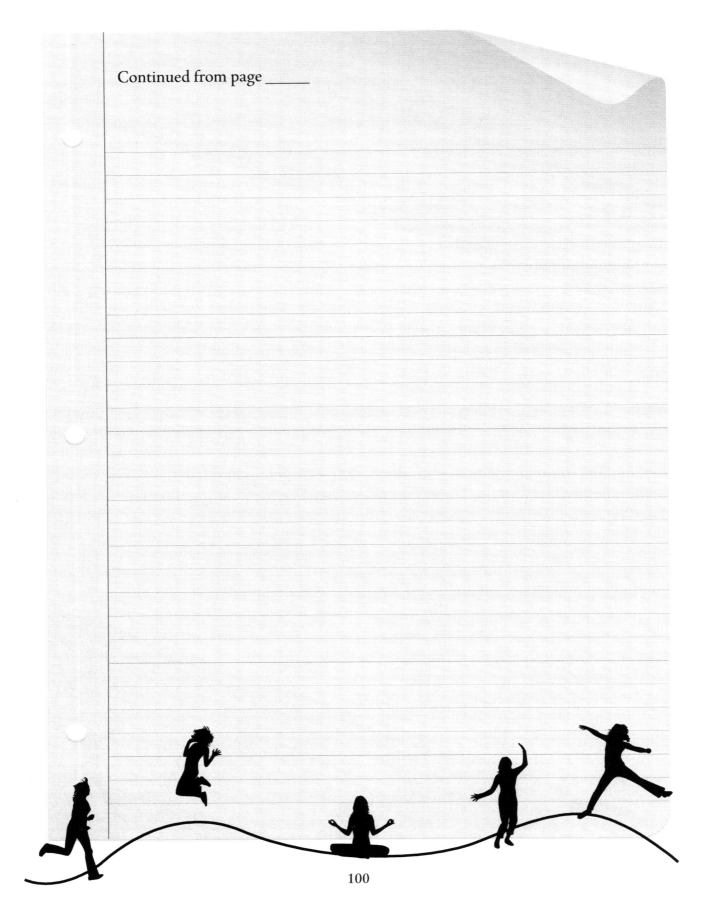

Continued from page _____

Continued from page _____

Continued from page _____

Made in the USA
Charleston, SC
14 June 2016